hatha yoga poses chart

HATHA YOGA POSES CHART CONTAINS 60 OF THE MOST COMMON BEGINNER AND INTERMEDIATE POSES, ORGANIZED INTO THE FOLLOWING SIX CATEGORIES: STANDING, SUPINE, SEATED, PRONE, KNEELING AND OTHER.

THE POSES ARE GROUPED BY ANATOMICAL POSITION SO THAT YOU CAN QUICKLY AND EASILY FIND THE POSE YOU'RE LOOKING FOR AS YOU PRACTICE.

THIS CHART CAN BE USED IN ONE, TWO OR ALL THREE OF THE FOLLOWING WAYS: MINI POSTER, BOOK, FLASH CARDS.

HOW TO USE

MINI POSTER – IF YOU WANT TO POST THIS CHART ON THE WALL, SIMPLY OPEN THE STAPLE IN THE MIDDLE OF THE BOOKLET AND REMOVE TWO PAGES THEN PIN TWO COPIES ON THE WALL (ONE FOR EACH SIDE).

BOOK – LEAVE ONE COPY IN THE BOOK AND STAND IT UP AS YOU DO YOUR YOGA PRACTICE OR USE IT AS A REFERENCE TO STUDY FROM OUTSIDE OF YOUR PRACTICE TIME.

FLASH CARDS – CUT THE FIGURES OUT AND MAKE FLASH CARDS OUT OF THEM.

© 2018 The Mindful Word, All rights reserved. Printed in the United States of America
The Mindful Word · 1120 Finch Ave. W. Unit 701-928, Toronto, Ontario, M3J 3H7, Canada
Visit us online at www.themindfulword.org

STANDING ASANAS

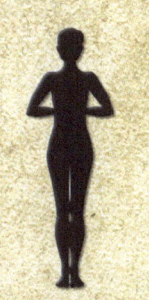
PRANAMASANA
Prayer Pose

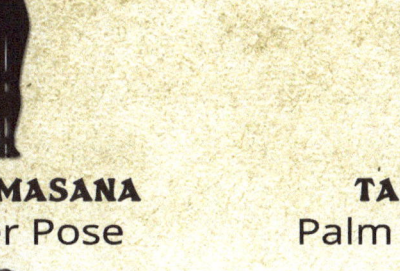
TALASANA
Palm Tree Pose

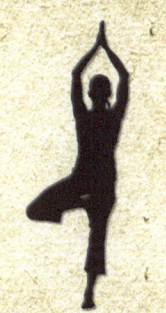
VRKSASANA
Tree Pose

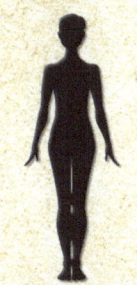
TADASANA
Mountain Pose

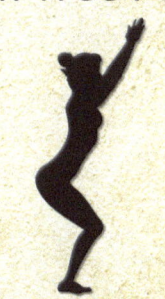
UTKATASANA
Chair Pose

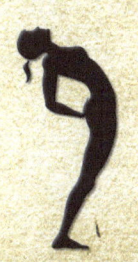
ANUVITTASANA
Standing Backbend Pose

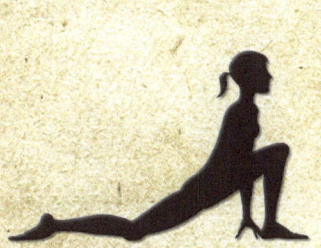
ANJANEYASANA
Low Lunge

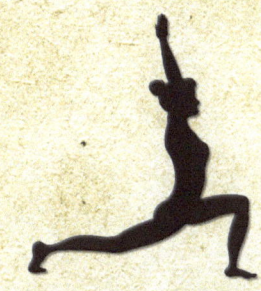
UTTHITA ASHWA SANCHALANASANA
High Lunge (Crescent Variation)

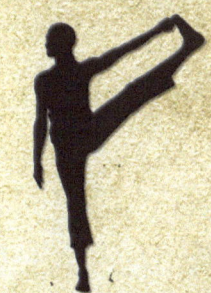
UTTHITA HASTA PADANGUSTASANA
Extended Hand-To-Big-Toe Pose

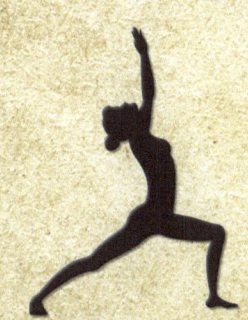
VIRABHADRASANA I
Warrior I Pose

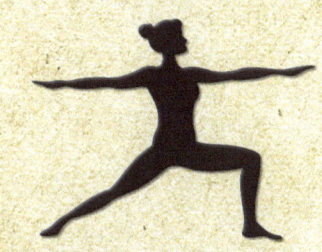
VIRABHADRASANA II
Warrior II Pose

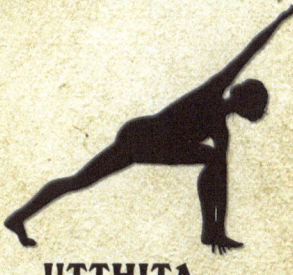
UTTHITA PARSVAKONASANA
Extended Side Angle Pose

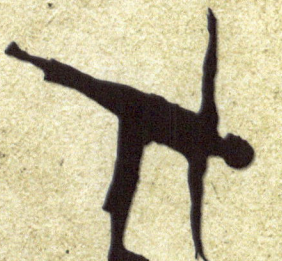
ARDHA CHANDRASANA
Half Moon Pose

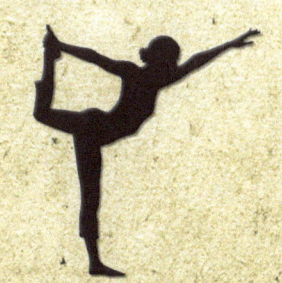
NATARAJASANA
Dancer's Pose

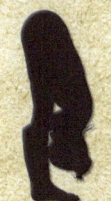
UTTANASANA
Standing Forward Bend

PRONE ASANAS

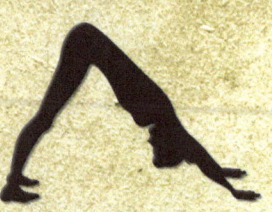
ADHO MUKHA SVANASANA
Downward-Facing Dog

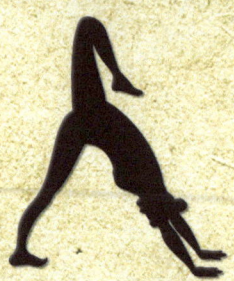
ADHO MUKHA SVANASANA
Downward-Facing Dog (variation)

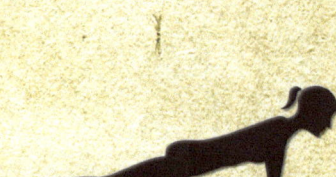
UTTANA SHISHOSANA
Extended Puppy Pose

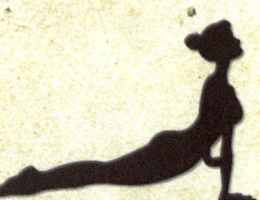
URDHVA MUKHA SVANASANA
Upward-Facing Dog

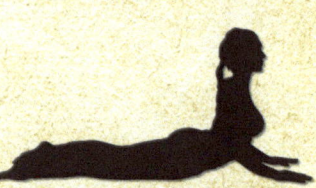
BHUJANGASANA
Cobra Pose

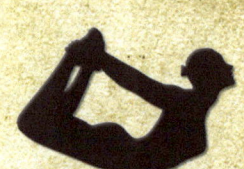
CHATURANGA DANDASANA
Four-Limbed Staff Pose

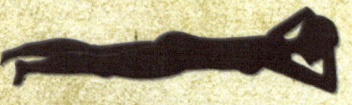
MAKARASANA
Crocodile Pose

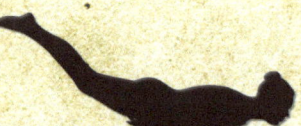
SALABHASANA
Locust Pose

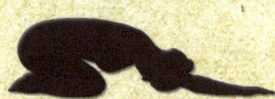
DHANURASANA
Bow Pose

KNEELING ASANAS

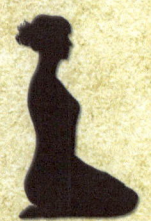
VAJRASANA
Thunderbolt Pose

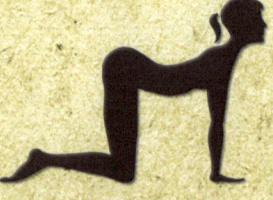
BALASANA
Child's Pose

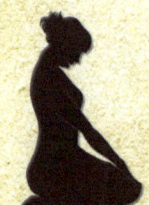
SIMHASANA
Lion Pose

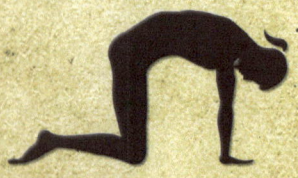
MARJARYASANA
Cat Pose

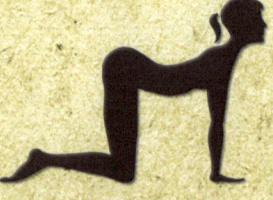
BITILASANA
Cow Pose

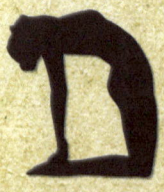
USTRASANA
Camel Pose

STANDING ASANAS

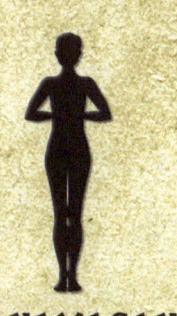
PRANAMASANA
Prayer Pose

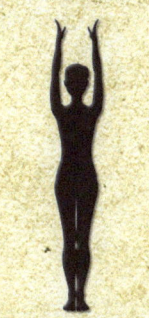
TALASANA
Palm Tree Pose

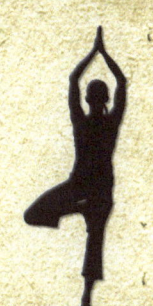
VRKSASANA
Tree Pose

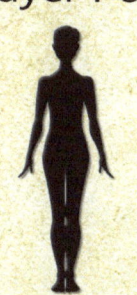
TADASANA
Mountain Pose

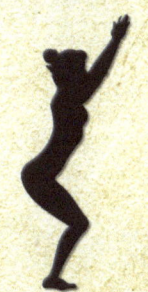
UTKATASANA
Chair Pose

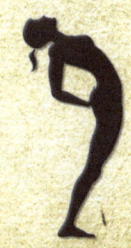
ANUVITTASANA
Standing Backbend Pose

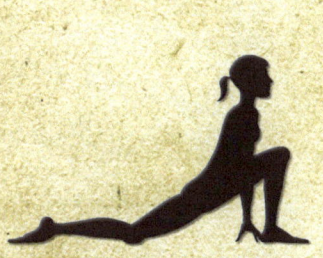
ANJANEYASANA
Low Lunge

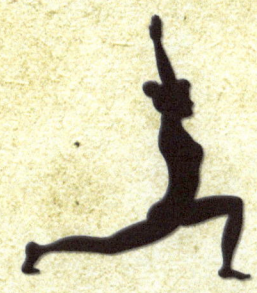
UTTHITA ASHWA SANCHALANASANA
High Lunge (Crescent Variation)

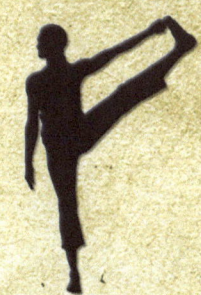
UTTHITA HASTA PADANGUSTASANA
Extended Hand-To-Big-Toe Pose

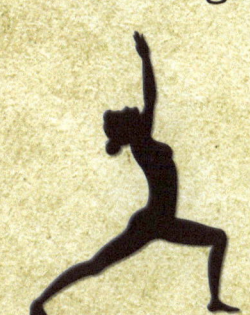
VIRABHADRASANA I
Warrior I Pose

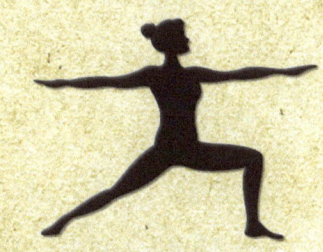
VIRABHADRASANA II
Warrior II Pose

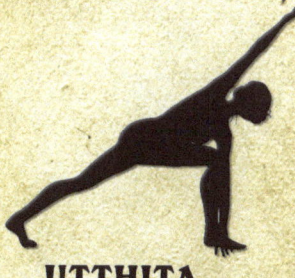
UTTHITA PARSVAKONASANA
Extended Side Angle Pose

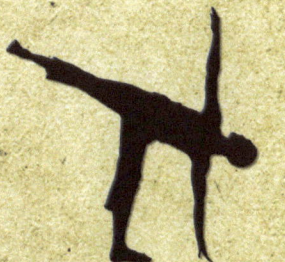
ARDHA CHANDRASANA
Half Moon Pose

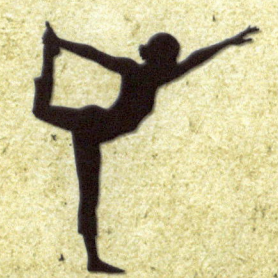
NATARAJASANA
Dancer's Pose

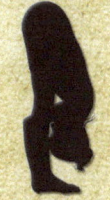
UTTANASANA
Standing Forward Bend

PRONE ASANAS

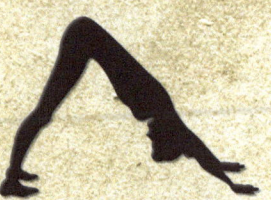
ADHO MUKHA SVANASANA
Downward-Facing Dog

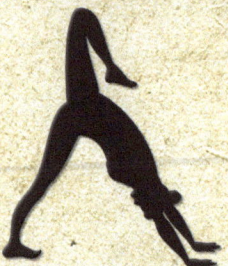
ADHO MUKHA SVANASANA
Downward-Facing Dog (variation)

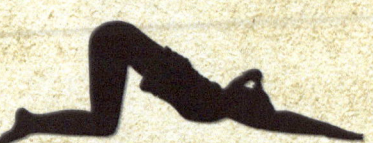
UTTANA SHISHOSANA
Extended Puppy Pose

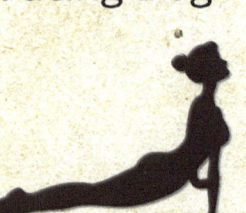
URDHVA MUKHA SVANASANA
Upward-Facing Dog

BHUJANGASANA
Cobra Pose

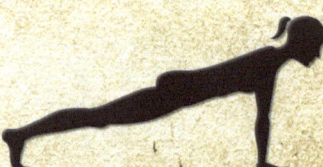
CHATURANGA DANDASANA
Four-Limbed Staff Pose

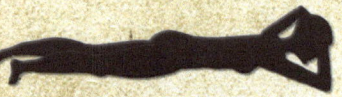
MAKARASANA
Crocodile Pose

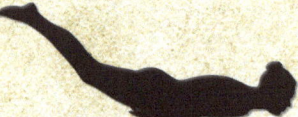
SALABHASANA
Locust Pose

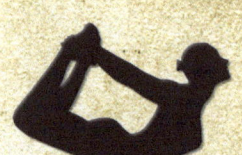
DHANURASANA
Bow Pose

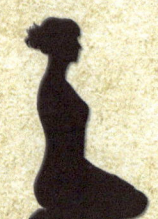
VAJRASANA
Thunderbolt Pose

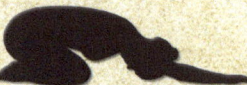
BALASANA
Child's Pose

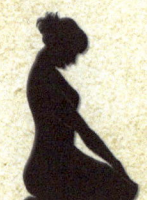
SIMHASANA
Lion Pose

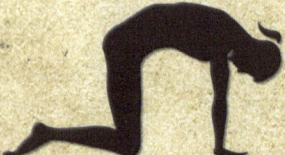
MARJARYASANA
Cat Pose

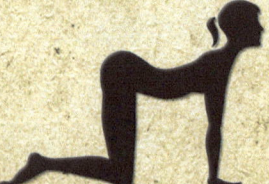
BITILASANA
Cow Pose

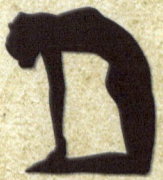
USTRASANA
Camel Pose

KNEELING ASANAS

STANDING ASANAS

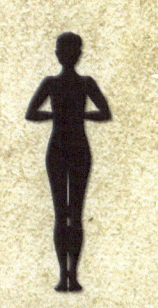
PRANAMASANA
Prayer Pose

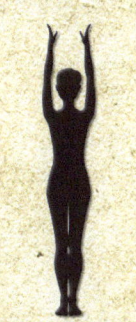
TALASANA
Palm Tree Pose

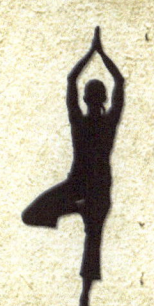
VRKSASANA
Tree Pose

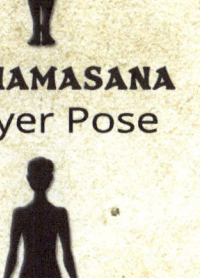
TADASANA
Mountain Pose

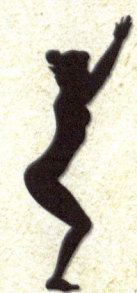
UTKATASANA
Chair Pose

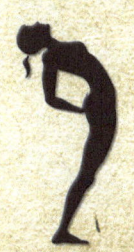
ANUVITTASANA
Standing Backbend Pose

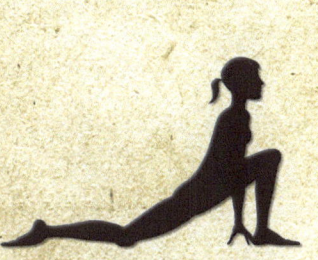
ANJANEYASANA
Low Lunge

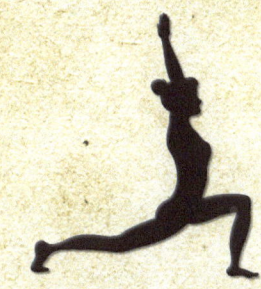
UTTHITA ASHWA SANCHALANASANA
High Lunge
(Crescent Variation)

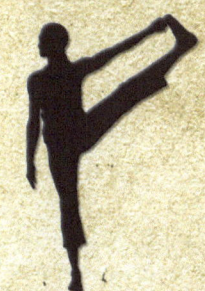
UTTHITA HASTA PADANGUSTASANA
Extended Hand-To-Big-Toe Pose

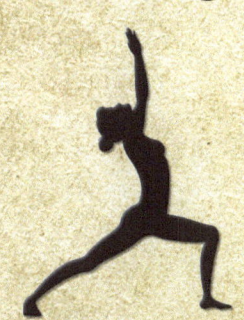
VIRABHADRASANA I
Warrior I Pose

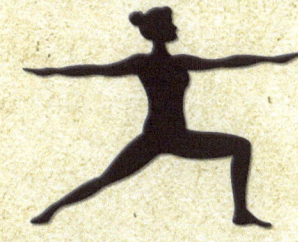
VIRABHADRASANA II
Warrior II Pose

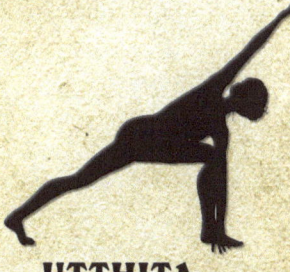
UTTHITA PARSVAKONASANA
Extended Side Angle Pose

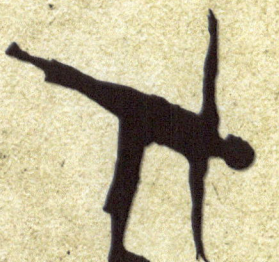
ARDHA CHANDRASANA
Half Moon Pose

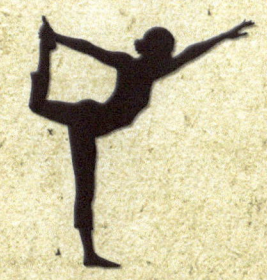
NATARAJASANA
Dancer's Pose

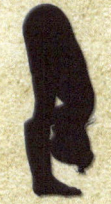
UTTANASANA
Standing Forward Bend

PRONE ASANAS

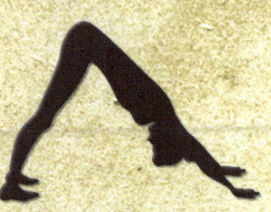
ADHO MUKHA SVANASANA
Downward-Facing Dog

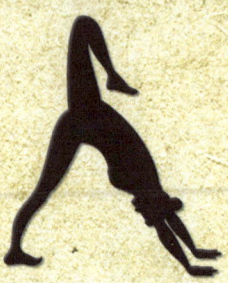
ADHO MUKHA SVANASANA
Downward-Facing Dog (variation)

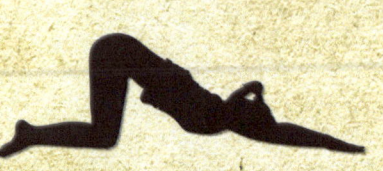
UTTANA SHISHOSANA
Extended Puppy Pose

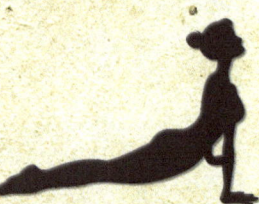
URDHVA MUKHA SVANASANA
Upward-Facing Dog

BHUJANGASANA
Cobra Pose

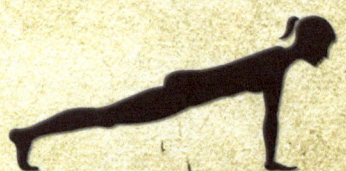
CHATURANGA DANDASANA
Four-Limbed Staff Pose

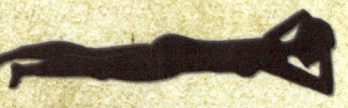
MAKARASANA
Crocodile Pose

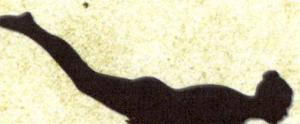
SALABHASANA
Locust Pose

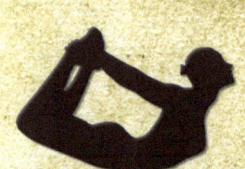
DHANURASANA
Bow Pose

KNEELING ASANAS

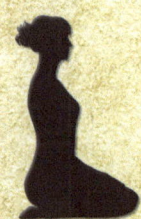
VAJRASANA
Thunderbolt Pose

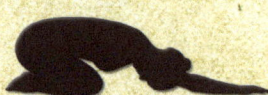
BALASANA
Child's Pose

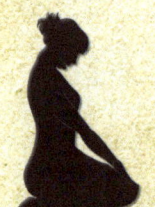
SIMHASANA
Lion Pose

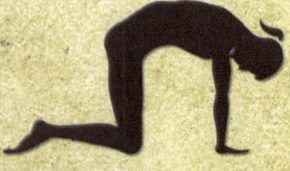
MARJARYASANA
Cat Pose

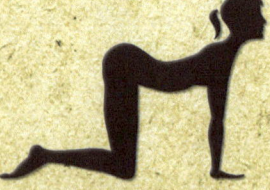
BITILASANA
Cow Pose

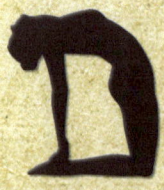
USTRASANA
Camel Pose

STANDING ASANAS

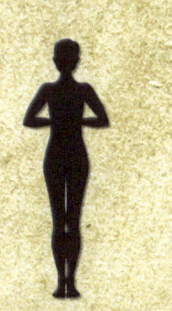
PRANAMASANA
Prayer Pose

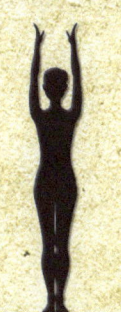
TALASANA
Palm Tree Pose

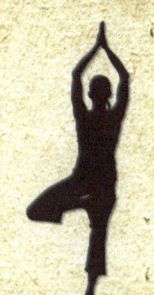
VRKSASANA
Tree Pose

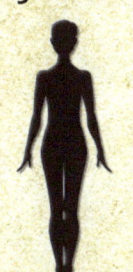
TADASANA
Mountain Pose

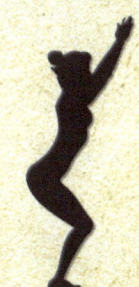
UTKATASANA
Chair Pose

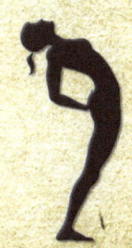
ANUVITTASANA
Standing Backbend Pose

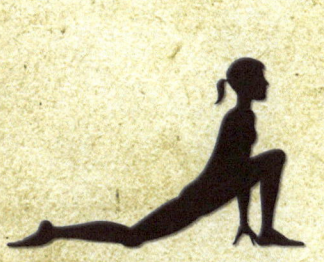
ANJANEYASANA
Low Lunge

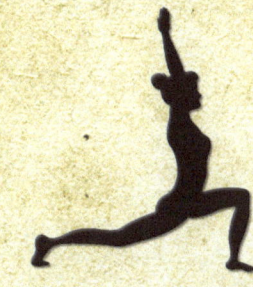
UTTHITA ASHWA SANCHALANASANA
High Lunge (Crescent Variation)

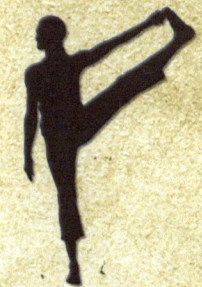
UTTHITA HASTA PADANGUSTASANA
Extended Hand-To-Big-Toe Pose

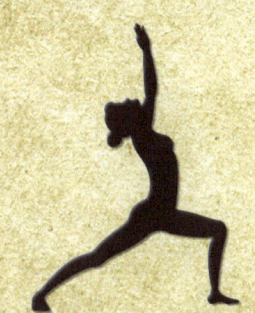
VIRABHADRASANA I
Warrior I Pose

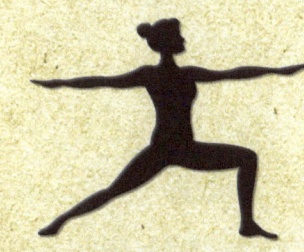
VIRABHADRASANA II
Warrior II Pose

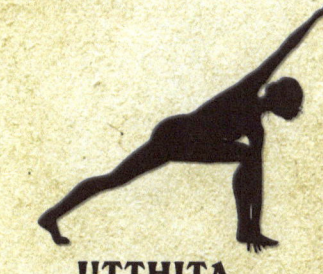
UTTHITA PARSVAKONASANA
Extended Side Angle Pose

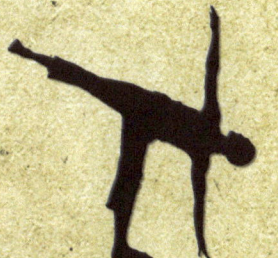
ARDHA CHANDRASANA
Half Moon Pose

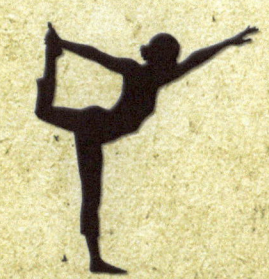
NATARAJASANA
Dancer's Pose

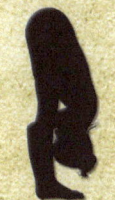
UTTANASANA
Standing Forward Bend

PRONE ASANAS

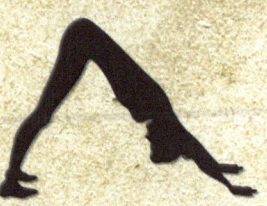
ADHO MUKHA SVANASANA
Downward-Facing Dog

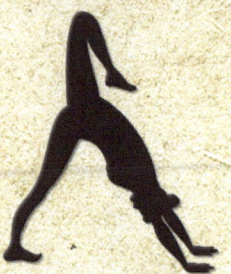
ADHO MUKHA SVANASANA
Downward-Facing Dog (variation)

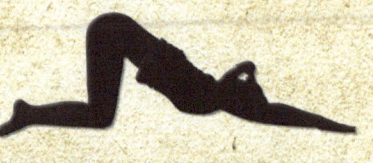
UTTANA SHISHOSANA
Extended Puppy Pose

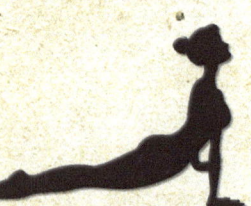
URDHVA MUKHA SVANASANA
Upward-Facing Dog

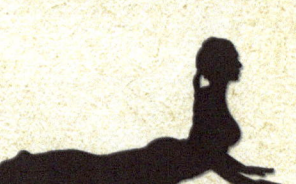
BHUJANGASANA
Cobra Pose

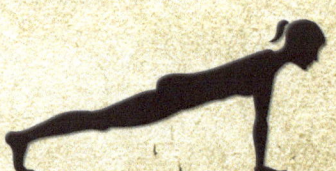
CHATURANGA DANDASANA
Four-Limbed Staff Pose

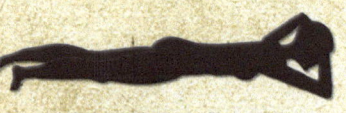
MAKARASANA
Crocodile Pose

SALABHASANA
Locust Pose

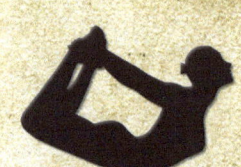
DHANURASANA
Bow Pose

KNEELING ASANAS

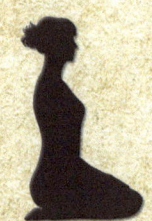
VAJRASANA
Thunderbolt Pose

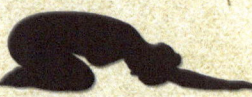
BALASANA
Child's Pose

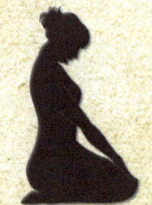
SIMHASANA
Lion Pose

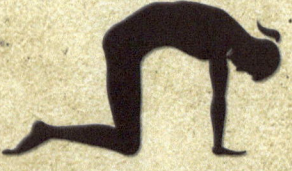
MARJARYASANA
Cat Pose

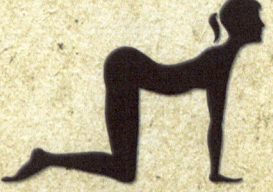
BITILASANA
Cow Pose

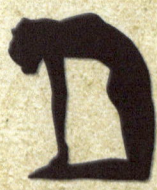
USTRASANA
Camel Pose

SEATED ASANAS

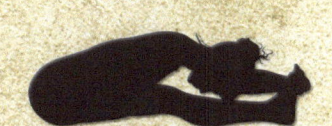
PASCHIMOTTANASANA
Seated Forward Bend

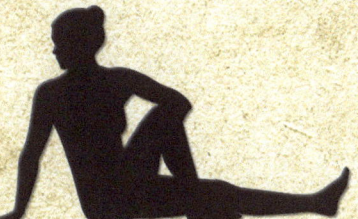
MARICHYASANA III
Marichi's Pose

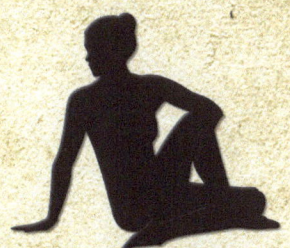
ARDHA MATYENDRASANA
Half Lord of the Fishes Pose

JANU SIRSASANA
Head-To-Knee Pose

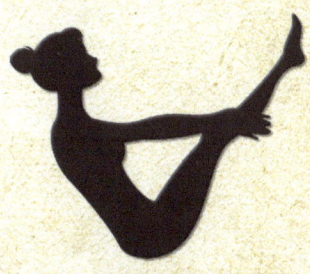
PARIPURNA NAVASANA
Boat Pose

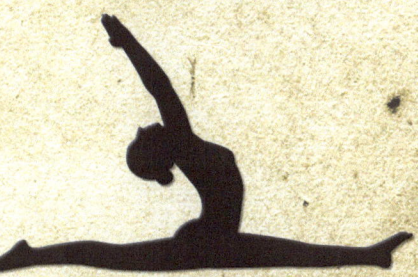
HANUMANASANA
Monkey Pose

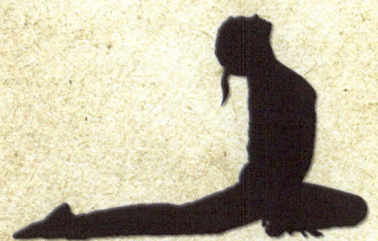
EKA PADA RAJAKAPOTASANA
Pigeon Pose

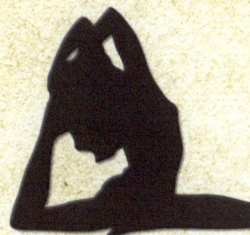
EKA PADA RAJAKAPOTASANA
Pigeon Pose (variation)

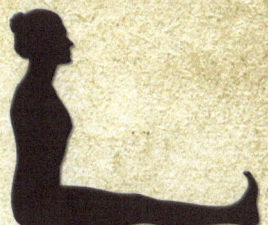
DANDASANA
Staff Pose

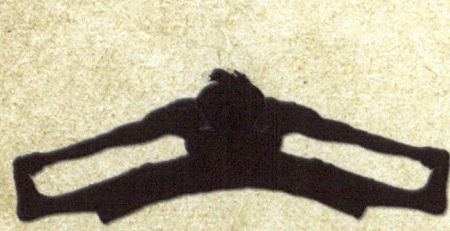
UPAVISTHA KONASANA
Wide-Angle Seated Forward Bend

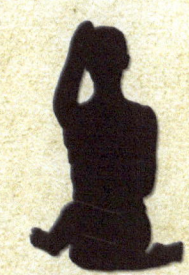
GOMUKHASANA
Cow Face Pose

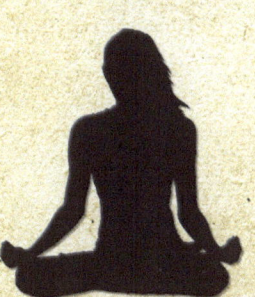
SVASTIKASANA
Cross Pose

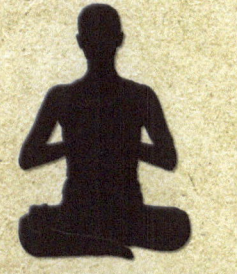
AGNISTAMBHASANA
Fire Log Pose

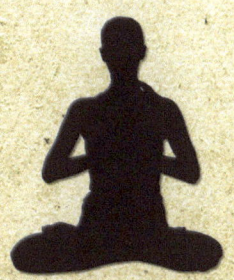
PADMASANA
Lotus Pose

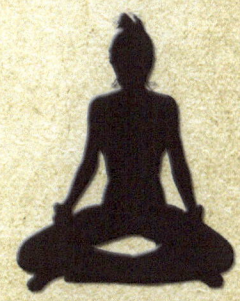
SUKHASANA
Easy Pose

SUPINE ASANAS

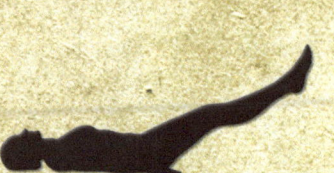
UTTANPADASANA
Raised-Leg Pose

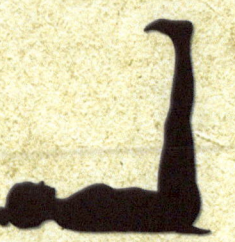
VIPARITA KARANI
Legs-Up-the-Wall Pose

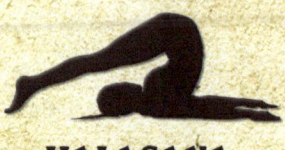
HALASANA
Plow Pose

PAVANAMUKTASANA
Wind Liberating Pose

MATSYASANA
Fish Pose

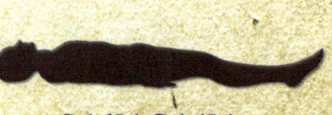
SAVASANA
Corpse Pose

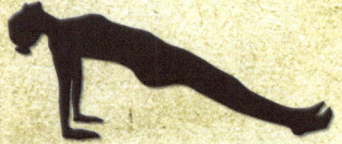
PURVOTTANASANA
Upward Plank Pose

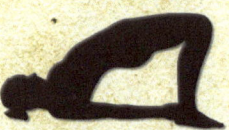
SETU BANDHA SARVANGASANA
Bridge Pose

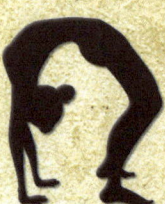
CHAKRASANA
Wheel Pose

OTHER ASANAS

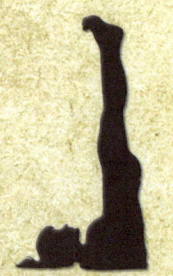
SARVANGASANA
Shoulderstand

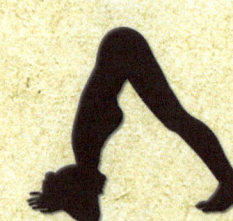
ARDHA SIRSASANA
Half Headstand

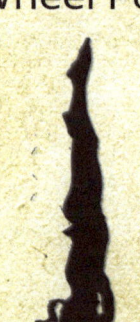
SIRSASANA
Headstand

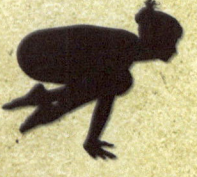
BAKASANA
Crow Pose

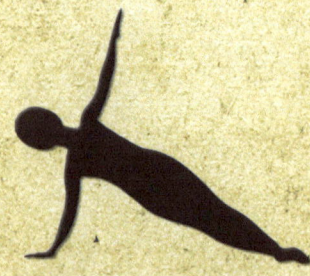
VASISTHASANA
Side Plank Pose

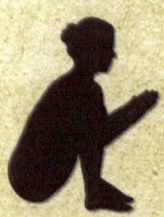
MALASANA
Garland Pose

SEATED ASANAS

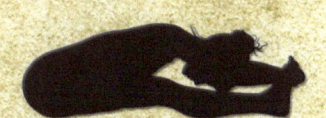
PASCHIMOTTANASANA
Seated Forward Bend

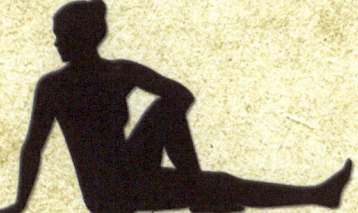
MARICHYASANA III
Marichi's Pose

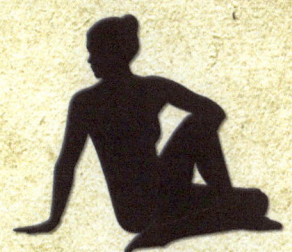
ARDHA MATYENDRASANA
Half Lord of the Fishes Pose

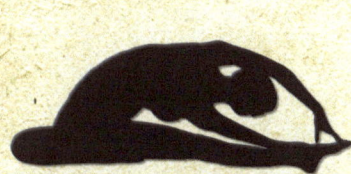
JANU SIRSASANA
Head-To-Knee Pose

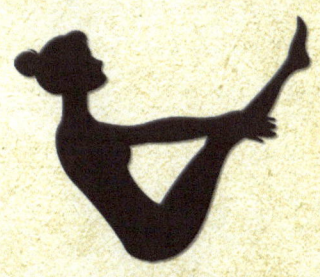
PARIPURNA NAVASANA
Boat Pose

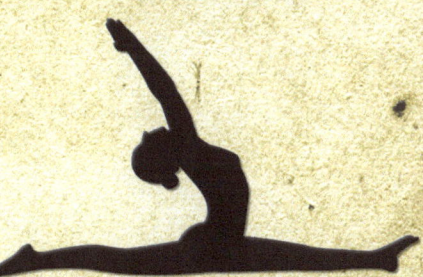
HANUMANASANA
Monkey Pose

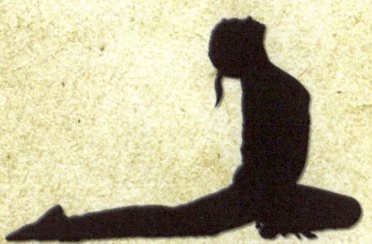
EKA PADA RAJAKAPOTASANA
Pigeon Pose

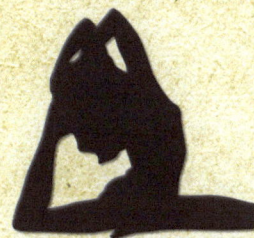
EKA PADA RAJAKAPOTASANA
Pigeon Pose (variation)

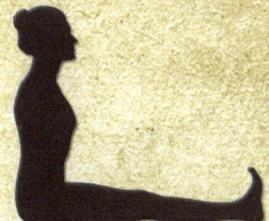
DANDASANA
Staff Pose

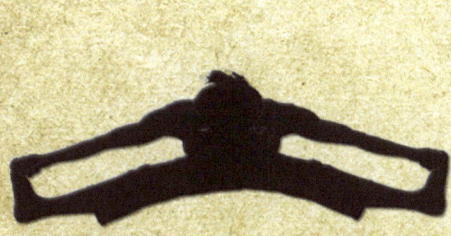
UPAVISTHA KONASANA
Wide-Angle Seated Forward Bend

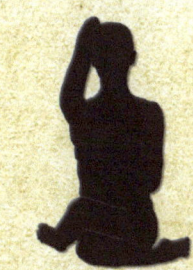
GOMUKHASANA
Cow Face Pose

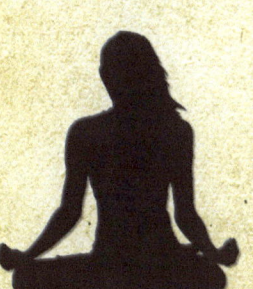
SVASTIKASANA
Cross Pose

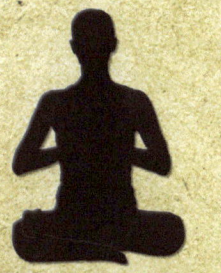
AGNISTAMBHASANA
Fire Log Pose

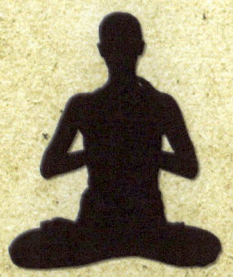
PADMASANA
Lotus Pose

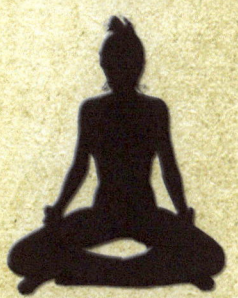
SUKHASANA
Easy Pose

SUPINE ASANAS

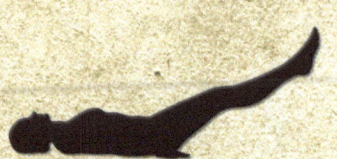
UTTANPADASANA
Raised-Leg Pose

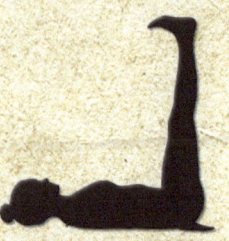
VIPARITA KARANI
Legs-Up-the-Wall Pose

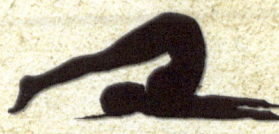
HALASANA
Plow Pose

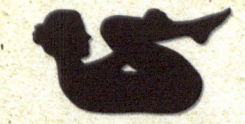
PAVANAMUKTASANA
Wind Liberating Pose

MATSYASANA
Fish Pose

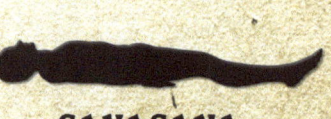
SAVASANA
Corpse Pose

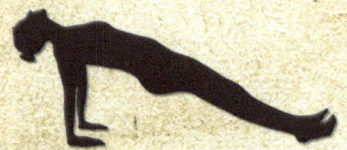
PURVOTTANASANA
Upward Plank Pose

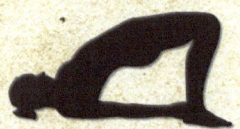
SETU BANDHA SARVANGASANA
Bridge Pose

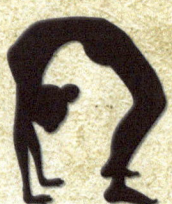
CHAKRASANA
Wheel Pose

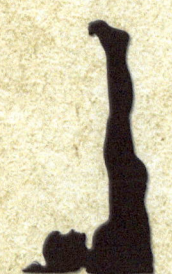
SARVANGASANA
Shoulderstand

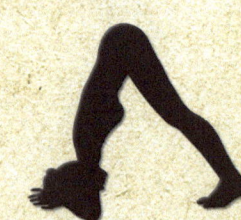
ARDHA SIRSASANA
Half Headstand

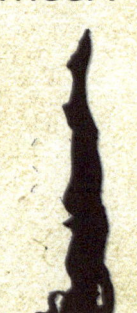
SIRSASANA
Headstand

OTHER ASANAS

BAKASANA
Crow Pose

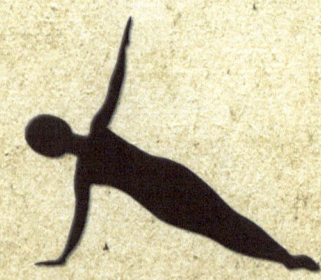
VASISTHASANA
Side Plank Pose

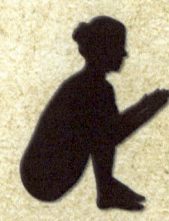
MALASANA
Garland Pose

SEATED ASANAS

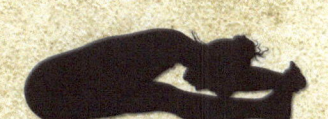
PASCHIMOTTANASANA
Seated Forward Bend

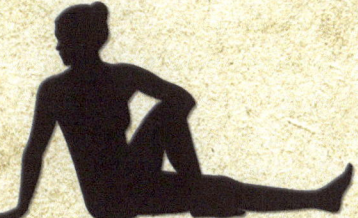
MARICHYASANA III
Marichi's Pose

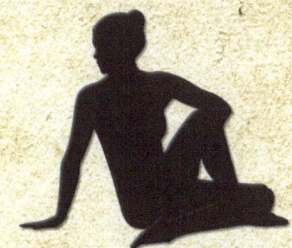
ARDHA MATYENDRASANA
Half Lord of the Fishes Pose

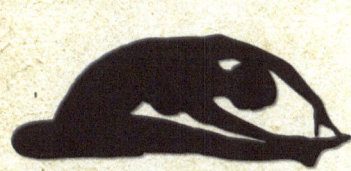
JANU SIRSASANA
Head-To-Knee Pose

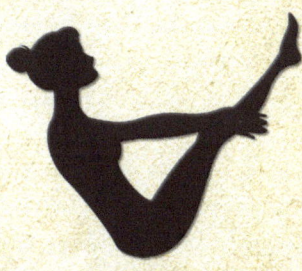
PARIPURNA NAVASANA
Boat Pose

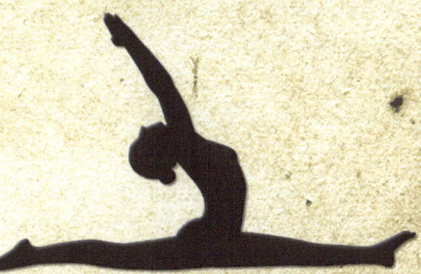
HANUMANASANA
Monkey Pose

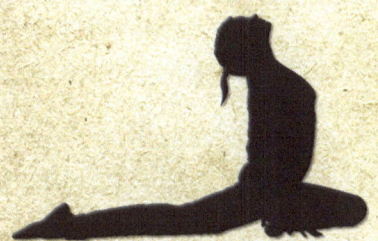
EKA PADA RAJAKAPOTASANA
Pigeon Pose

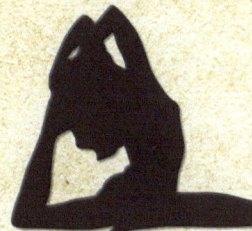
EKA PADA RAJAKAPOTASANA
Pigeon Pose (variation)

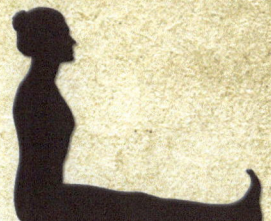
DANDASANA
Staff Pose

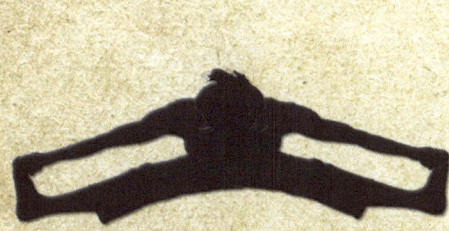
UPAVISTHA KONASANA
Wide-Angle Seated Forward Bend

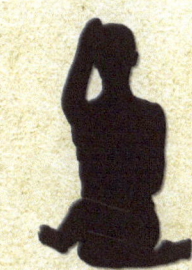
GOMUKHASANA
Cow Face Pose

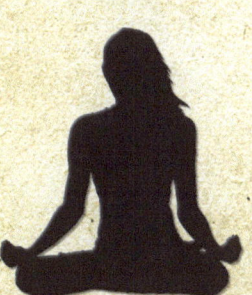
SVASTIKASANA
Cross Pose

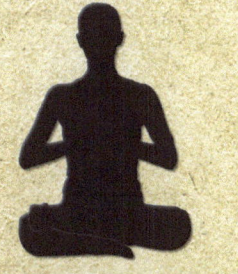
AGNISTAMBHASANA
Fire Log Pose

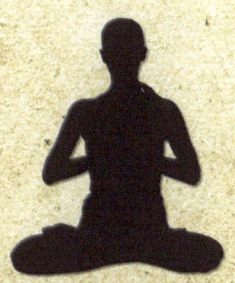
PADMASANA
Lotus Pose

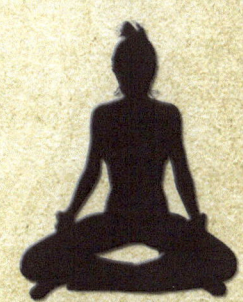
SUKHASANA
Easy Pose

SUPINE ASANAS | **OTHER ASANAS**

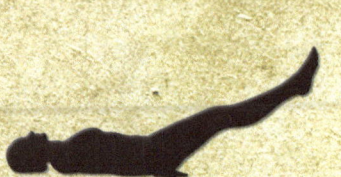
UTTANPADASANA
Raised-Leg Pose

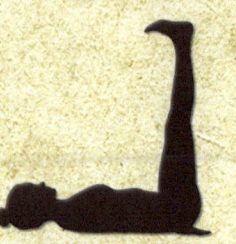
VIPARITA KARANI
Legs-Up-the-Wall Pose

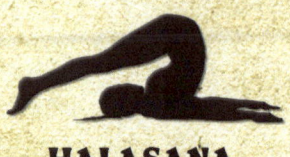
HALASANA
Plow Pose

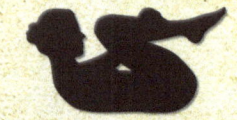
PAVANAMUKTASANA
Wind Liberating Pose

MATSYASANA
Fish Pose

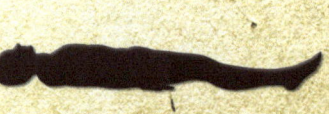
SAVASANA
Corpse Pose

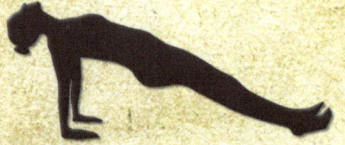
PURVOTTANASANA
Upward Plank Pose

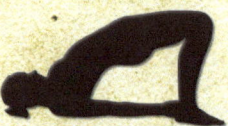
SETU BANDHA SARVANGASANA
Bridge Pose

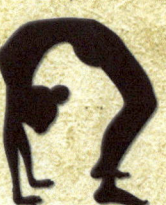
CHAKRASANA
Wheel Pose

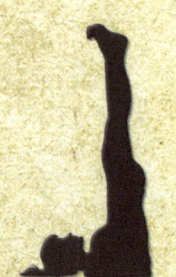
SARVANGASANA
Shoulderstand

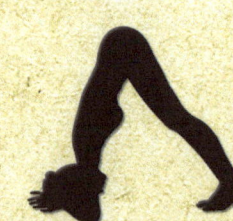
ARDHA SIRSASANA
Half Headstand

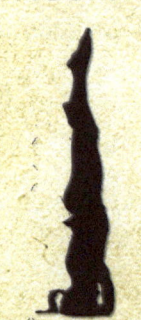
SIRSASANA
Headstand

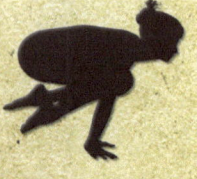
BAKASANA
Crow Pose

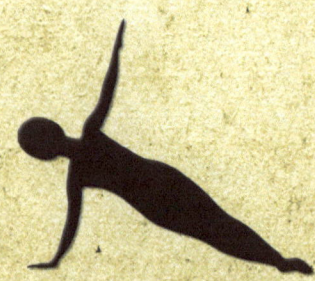
VASISTHASANA
Side Plank Pose

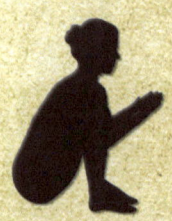
MALASANA
Garland Pose

SEATED ASANAS

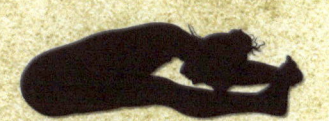
PASCHIMOTTANASANA
Seated Forward Bend

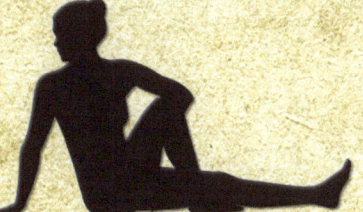
MARICHYASANA III
Marichi's Pose

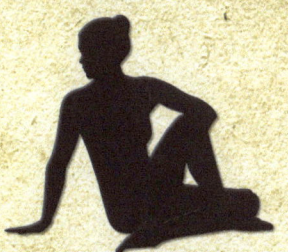
ARDHA MATYENDRASANA
Half Lord of the Fishes Pose

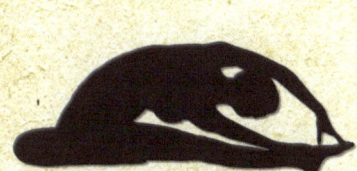
JANU SIRSASANA
Head-To-Knee Pose

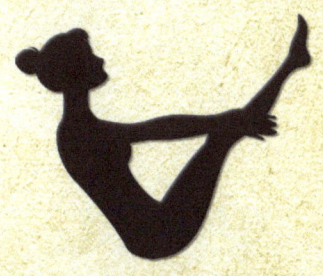
PARIPURNA NAVASANA
Boat Pose

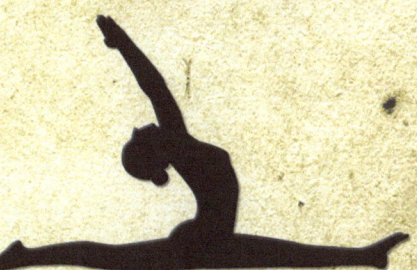
HANUMANASANA
Monkey Pose

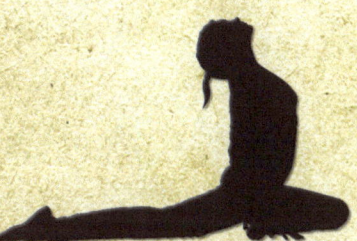
EKA PADA RAJAKAPOTASANA
Pigeon Pose

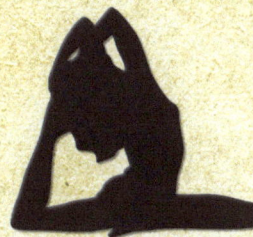
EKA PADA RAJAKAPOTASANA
Pigeon Pose (variation)

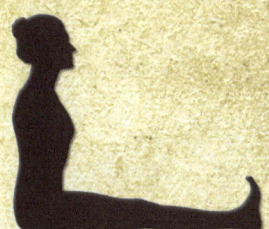
DANDASANA
Staff Pose

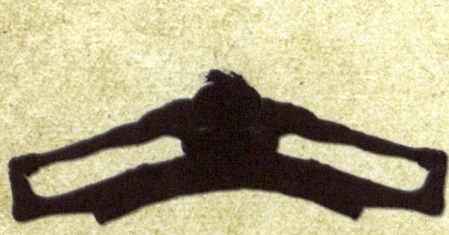
UPAVISTHA KONASANA
Wide-Angle Seated Forward Bend

GOMUKHASANA
Cow Face Pose

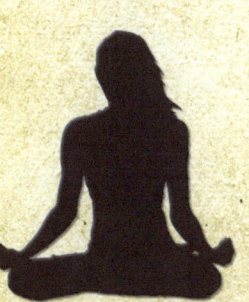
SVASTIKASANA
Cross Pose

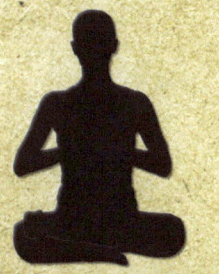
AGNISTAMBHASANA
Fire Log Pose

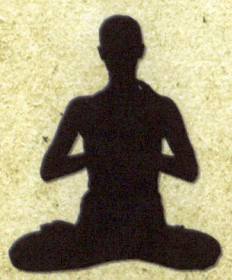
PADMASANA
Lotus Pose

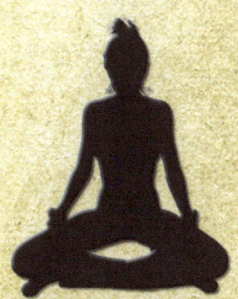
SUKHASANA
Easy Pose

SUPINE ASANAS

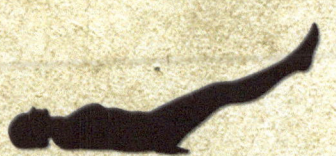
UTTANPADASANA
Raised-Leg Pose

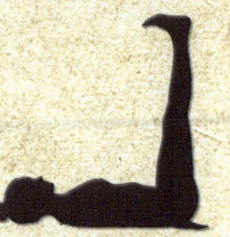
VIPARITA KARANI
Legs-Up-the-Wall Pose

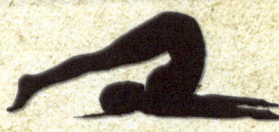
HALASANA
Plow Pose

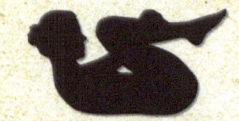
PAVANAMUKTASANA
Wind Liberating Pose

MATSYASANA
Fish Pose

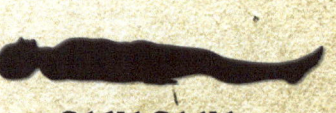
SAVASANA
Corpse Pose

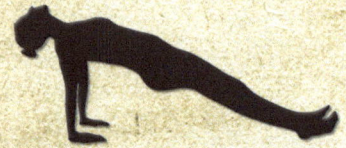
PURVOTTANASANA
Upward Plank Pose

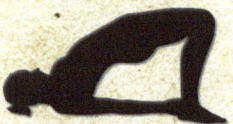
SETU BANDHA SARVANGASANA
Bridge Pose

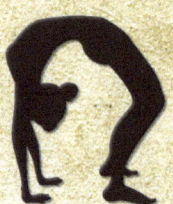
CHAKRASANA
Wheel Pose

OTHER ASANAS

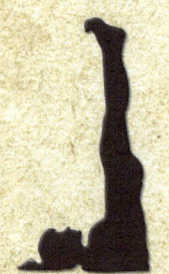
SARVANGASANA
Shoulderstand

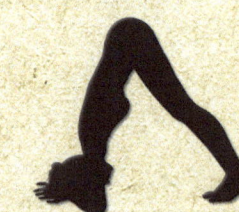
ARDHA SIRSASANA
Half Headstand

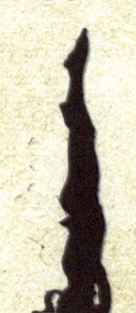
SIRSASANA
Headstand

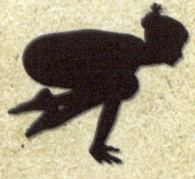
BAKASANA
Crow Pose

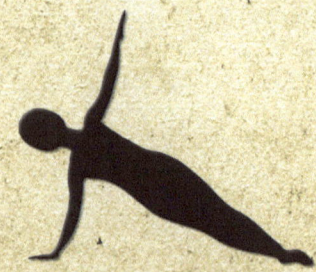
VASISTHASANA
Side Plank Pose

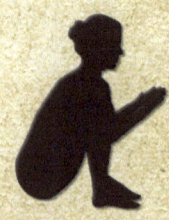
MALASANA
Garland Pose

www.ingramcontent.com/pod-product-compliance
Lightning Source LLC
Chambersburg PA
CBHW040440040426

42333CB00034B/46